Cheat Sheet

Weight loss goal _____ kg
Weeks to lose weight _____ weeks
BMR _____ calories
Maintenance calories _____ calories
Lean Body Mass (LBM) _____ kg

Diet calories _____ calories

Protein _____ grams _____ calories _____ %
Carbs _____ grams _____ calories _____ %
Fats _____ grams _____ calories _____ %

Carb refeed _____ grams _____ calories

Other titles by **SHARNY & JULIUS**

Never Diet Again: Escape the diet trap forever

Fit, Healthy, Happy Mum: How my quest for perfect breastmilk helped me lose 24 kilos in only 8 weeks after the birth of my fourth child

FITlosophy 1: Chasing physical perfection in the world of gluttony

FITlosophy 2: Expanding perfection against the rise of OOC

Healthy JUNK: Healthy versions of your favorite junk foods

Healthy JUNK 2: 50 more guilt-free delicious recipes

Fit, Healthy, Happy Kids: A food and exercise blueprint for children under 12

Fertile: Understanding babymaking

PregFit: How I finally had a fit, healthy, happy pregnancy and pain-free birth

Where Have All The Pixies Gone?

THE MATH DIET

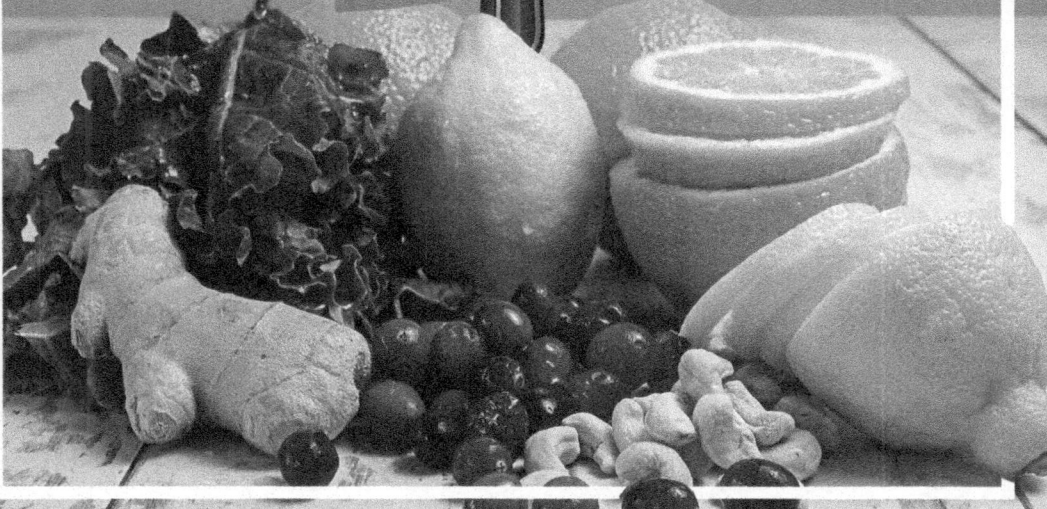

The simple step by step guide to Carb Cycling

SHARNY & JULIUS
www.sharnyandjulius.com

The Math Diet by SHARNY & JULIUS
You deserve to know

www.sharnyandjulius.com
email:sharnyandjulius@sharnyandjulius.com

Copyright © the Kieser Publishing Trust
First published by Kieser Publishing Trust in May 2015

The moral rights of the authors have been asserted. The stories, suggestions and opinions of the authors are their personal views only, and they are simply that, just stories, not historical accounts. The strategies and steps outlined in the book may not work for everyone. Due diligence and thorough research is always recommended.

All rights reserved. This book may not be reproduced in whole or in part, stored, posted on the internet or transmitted in any form or by any means, electronic, mechanical, photocopying, recording, or other, without written permission from the Authors and publisher of the book.

Edited by:	Laura Johnson
Cover Photography:	sharnyandjulius
Typesetting and Design:	sharnyandjulius
ISBN:	978-0-9923613-5-8

Contents

How to use this book	7
How much and by when?	9
Concepts are not diets	11
Commercial diets	17
The biggest secret	21
How long will it take?	23
You, in a coma	27
How your lifestyle computes	35
Bonus: Breastfeeding	39
Check it	41
How long will it take me?	43
How to estimate your body fat percentage	47
How to prevent muscle loss	51
Fats	59
Macronutrient balancing	65
How to eat whatever you want	69
Prioritise health	73
How to lose the first few kilos really fast	77
How to never be hungry	81
Avoid starvation mode	89
Increase your metabolism	95
Putting it all together	99

How to use this book

Think of this book as a workbook, we have included plenty of space for notes and for calculations. If math makes your hands sweat, don't worry. The maths that you will do is so basic that a primary school child can do it.

All you'll need to get the most out of this book is a pencil and the calculator on your phone. Please don't be afraid to write all through the book - it's designed to be used like a workbook. The more you write the more you will get out of this book.

The chapters are set out in a logical, step by step process. Try not to skip ahead, as you may miss out on an important calculation. You'll notice in the very front of the book, we have included a cheat sheet to keep all of your most important numbers. As you go through the book, fill this out because you'll need to refer to these numbers often. To make it even easier, we'll tell you when one of these numbers comes up.

Enjoy the book, even if you never liked maths in school, the simple use of it in this book will give you insight into your life that you never thought possible before!

How much and by when?

In this book, we're going to teach you exactly how to lose weight, not by some wishy washy concept, or by using some proprietary points counting thing you have to pay for.

Throughout this book, you will be given the tools to be able to control your own body composition. Tools that until now have been the reserve of champion body builders, fitness models and high end physique coaches.

We're not saying "hey, do this and you'll lose a bunch of weight…" That's bullshit and plain rude. *How much and by when?* Nobody tells you how much and by when. Why? Well, for two reasons – firstly, because they have no idea. It's much easier to say, "you'll lose some weight doing this," than to give you an exact amount, a time frame and a why.

Secondly, it admonishes them and you of responsibility. "If it doesn't work, then well, try *this*…"

We won't do that to you. You deserve to know exactly how much weight you will lose, by when and most importantly, *why*. We don't like the idea of knowing the answer and keeping it a secret from you, even if it means you coming back to us, time and time again. We'll leave that to the big commercial diet companies whose primary objective is your wallet.

In fact, you'll work through this book and wonder why you never knew this. It's not difficult, it's actually very, very easy. But don't let the ease of it fool you, this is very powerful stuff.

Concepts are not diets

How do you know somebody is Vegan?
*Don't worry, they'll f***ng tell you.*

There are two types of diets. Conceptual diets, and commercial diets. We'll touch on commercial diets in the next chapter, but for now, let's look at conceptual (fad) diets.

Conceptual diets are exactly that, concepts. They can be recognised by having broad rules about what you can or can't eat. They can more easily be recognised by their followers. Like religious fanatics, the most passionate of them will be near foaming at the mouth to tell you how great they feel. Like religious fanatics, their way is the only way, everything else is just a fad.

Examples of conceptual diets include Paleo, Vegan, Vegetarian, Low Fat, Banting, Sugar Free and many other fad diets that come and go.

The problem with using concepts as diets is that concepts can be manipulated. Think about Paleo for a moment, we can all agree that Paleo is the biggest concept diet on the market today. Paleo works, it stops people from eating junk food. Eating whole foods is much better than pies and soft drink... But it doesn't take a scientist to see that in Paleo's short life it has already been manipulated and bastardised into a Frankenstein of a concept.

Walk into a paleo restaurant and look at the menu – nothing on there resembles food a cave man would eat. Now, we're no experts, but we're pretty sure cavemen didn't have blenders. Cavemen didn't know how to cold press coconut oil, extract ghee from the local yak and mix a tablespoon of each into a shot of Arabica coffee he'd prepared…

Concepts can be manipulated.

The other thing you may notice about conceptual diets is that they tend to cut out one or two macronutrients. The trouble with this approach is that when you don't balance your macronutrients (more on this later), the one that is left out gets really, really agitated. If you've ever consciously cut out carbs, you'll know what we mean.

Almost immediately you miss carbs. You start saying things like "I wonder how anyone survives without them." You start to see carbs everywhere, and when you sleep, all you can dream about is carbs. Your stomach yearns for them. You fight these thoughts, telling yourself that it's just a detox phase, it will go away.

One day the natural yearning for carbs becomes too much and you find yourself sitting in the bottom of the pantry, surrounded by wrappers, stomach stretched, lips glistening, thinking about all the other times you've failed at life.

We are teasing a bit here. Conceptual diets are not bad, they're usually the starting point for people trying to get healthy. If it takes a thesis on human evolution for someone to realise that junk food is not good for them, then we're all for it.

That's just it though, eating healthy is so easy that it's just not cool. Far more interesting to have some vague link to a time period than to just say "I just don't eat junk."

Concepts come and go, like fashion. People get some results and tell everyone about this new miracle way of eating. "I'm Paleo," they say. "It's this eating style where you eat just like a caveman. It just makes my body sing, it's giving me life back and I feel amazing!"

"Oh, I did that caveman style, but I'm doing Banting now. Basically I just eat fat and nothing else. My skin is glowing and I haven't slept so well in years. It's the newest thing. You should try it, cavemen were so last century, polar bears are where it's at this year."

We're teasing again, but here's a serious question for all the conceptual diet aficionados – did you get results from your concept because it's the greatest eating style ever created, or because it was just better than what you were eating before?

Here's another question. How much fat will I lose on your diet and how long will it take?

Concepts are mostly about health, with the side effect of weight loss. How much you lose is unknowable, you just get what you're given. Most of it is actually inflammation from your previous eating style.

A conceptual diet should be thought of as an eating style, not a diet. A diet should have a start, a finish and should be measurable.

We're not arguing the health benefits of concepts. Keep your concept in your pocket, because you can actually plug it into the Math Diet framework. What we're saying is that a *diet* should be about health *and* fat loss.

Commercial diets

*"You can check out any time you like,
but you can never leave."*

Commercial diets work. They work because they are mathematical. People get results from Jenny Craig and Weight Watchers, no doubt. The are diets, because they have a start, a finish and are measurable. They are not fashionable, but they work. They are not without their flaws though.

There's a reason they are such big companies… they keep secrets. They make sure that your money keeps going to them. You are a cash machine to them. You've got no self control, so you've got to come back… *ka-ching!* You've got to eat certain foods, we've got you covered there, just buy anything that has our logo on it… *ka-ching!* Or, "here's a book where we've made the counting really easy for you, because you're so dumb. It's got numbers, you just have to eat up to this number every day." *ka-ching!*

Worst of all is the company that sells you their chemical shitstorm of a shake. "It's got everything you need to replace a meal." Other than nutrition and a feeling of fullness.

Once you walk into a Commercial Diet, you're walking into their world, where everything is available to you, if you hand over your wallet and control of your life... And if you stay forever... Commercial diets are like Hotel California. You can check out any time you like, but you can never leave.

So we'll revise our analysis. Commercial diets have a start, are measurable but have no real end. Because even when you get to your goal weight, you still need to eat food with their logo on it, use their points counting system, or pay for their advice to make sure you never gain the weight back…

Wouldn't it be great if you knew what the mega commercial diet companies knew so that you could eat any food you liked, even if it didn't have their label on it?

Well, we're going to teach you, and it's not that complicated. In fact, it's quite easy and once you get it, it will be the most powerful lesson in your life. Because knowing your numbers is one of the most empowering freeing feelings you can ever have. Even more than that time you did a budget.

If you've never done a budget, we encourage you to do one. You may not think you need to, but immediately after finishing your budget, you get this overwhelming feeling of power, of self control. You stand up and you say to yourself, "I got this." Pride beams from you because you have actually worked out how and when you'll get your debt paid off, or how and when you're going to save for that holiday.

Throughout this book, you'll get that feeling. If, before you bought this book, you thought you were at the mercy of food companies and diet companies, rest easy. We've got the key here to the CEO's safe. Where all the secrets are kept.

Come inside.

We're going to show you exactly how much you can lose, how long it's going to take, how to do it, how to stay accountable… and it's not going to cost you a thing.

The biggest secret

We're going to let you in on the biggest secret of all. Once you've read this you're going to wonder why you never knew. Once you know this one little secret, you're going to be infinitely better off in your life.

The secret is that there are 9 calories per gram of fat. Some of you may already know this about food. Hell, we knew this for 10 years before it clicked.

Here's the distinction, fat is fat, whether it is in your food, or *on your body*.

We'll go further. If there are 9 calories per gram and there are 1,000 grams per kilo. That means there are 9,000 calories per kilo of fat. Let us make this even clearer. You need to burn 9,000 calories to lose one kilo of fat. Or, you need to eat 9,000 calories less than normal to lose one kilo of fat.

Why is this important? It's not just important, it's essential! Essential to giving you an honest expectation.

9,000 calories is a LOT! Most people use between 1,800 and 3,000 calories per day. Even at the top end, it would take 3 days of starvation nothing at all to lose a single kilo of fat. That's assuming the body doesn't do what it always does and take energy from stored carbs and muscle, and at the same time downregulate your metabolism.

9,000 calories is a lot. Fat loss requires *patience*. Most bodybuilders do a cut (fat loss diet) that lasts 3-6 months, and they're *already lean*.

Throw out any idea or book or friend that even hints at fast results. Yes, get the results as fast as you can, but don't be fooled into believing that you can lose *fat* fast. You can lose *weight* fast, and we'll teach you how to do that later in the book, but the weight you're losing isn't only fat.

Note: Even though food labelling has kJ and not calories, most of the world still uses calories. To convert kJ to calories, just divide by 4.18

_____kJ ÷ 4.18 = _____Cal

_____Cal x 4.18 = _____kJ

e.g. 9,000 Cal x 4.18 = 37,620 kJ

How long will it take?

So for you, let's get your expectation right now. This means getting out a pencil and a calculator. Your phone's calculator is fine, the sums are pretty simple.

How many kilos of fat do you want to lose?
To convert lbs to kg, just divide your lbs by 2.2 e.g.: 33lb / 2.2 = 15kg

Write your answer in here:

I want to lose _____ kg

Multiply the number you wrote down by 2.57. This is how many weeks it will take to lose the weight with a 500 calorie per day deficit.

_____ kg x 2.57 = _____ weeks.

e.g. 15 x 2.57 = 38.5 weeks. This means it will take 38 and a half weeks to lose 15kg at a 500 calorie per day deficit.

If you think you can handle a higher daily deficit, we'll calculate what how long it would take at a 1,000 calorie daily deficit. Just multiply the kilos of fat you want to lose by 1.29

_____ kg x 1.29 = _____ weeks

Sticking with our example of 15kg, it would take 15 x 1.29 = 19 weeks to lose 15kg at a 1,000 calorie per day deficit.

A 1,000 calorie deficit is really, really big. It's noticeable. You'll feel hungry and your body will respond. If your maintenance calories are 2,000, then that means you have to eat half of what you normally eat for at least 19 weeks. 19 weeks is over 4 months. A whole season. Chances are you're reading this book because you've been eating *more* than your maintenance calories.

So let's say you're used to eating 3,000 calories. You will therefore have to drop 2,000 calories a day, which means for at least 4 months, you have to eat a third of what you're used to.

Use this to give yourself a realistic expectation. We'll go into exact figures as we progress through the book, but we just wanted to show you how long it really takes. There's no arguing with this, there's no "miracle weight loss" or fast fat loss. It's all mathematical.

This calculation may be disheartening, but the good news is that now you know. Now you know how long it will take. And 4 months isn't that long. Hell, 2 years isn't that long if you actually get there.

Time is also relative, let us show you.

If we were to say that you needed to eat 1,000 calories less per day for 12 weeks so that you can lose 10kg, you'd probably feel like it's a long time, right? Well, what if we said that if you ate 1,000 calories more than you need, you'll be 10kg heavier in only 12 weeks. That sounds like a very short time, right?

Because it's mathematical, it comes on and off at the same rate, it's just that it's so much easier to eat 1,000 extra calories, and it's actually enjoyable. It's not that easy to eat 1,000 calories less, and it's not enjoyable.

But, just like every other person on earth who needed to lose weight, you got yourself into this situation, so you've got to get yourself out. The sooner you start, the sooner it will be over. The exciting thing is that the results happen immediately. Lucky for you it's not like jail, where you have to wait to the end of your sentence. You start losing weight straight away and you'll see changes every single week.

You, in a coma

In the previous chapter, we spoke about *maintenance calories*. Maintenance is a really important concept to understand, and like the 9,000 calories per kilo of fat, it gives you another critical key of knowledge that you just can't ever lose.

A calorie is a unit of energy. Like a centimetre is a measurement of distance, or a second is a measurement of time. A calorie is actually measured by heat. So when we say how many calories you burn a day, we literally mean burn, because each cell in your body is like a little fire that burns fat, carbs and/or protein to do stuff.

When we talk about your maintenance calories, what we mean is how many calories you burn each day. Adding up all the energy used by all the little fires in a 24 hour period.

By knowing how many calories you burn, we can know how many calories you need to replace the burnt energy. The coolest thing of all is that we know how much energy is stored in pretty much every food on earth. In fact, it's a legal requirement of food manufacturers to find out and to tell you.

Food labels are there to tell us that "for 100g of this food, you will get X amount of calories."

All the little cells in your body use energy. That energy has to come from somewhere. There are only two places it can come from; food, or stored food.

If you ate just enough food that your body didn't have to tap into stored food, then you ate your maintenance calories. It is the number of calories required to maintain your current body composition. If you ate your maintenance calories, you would not put on fat, nor would you lose it.

This number is as unique as your fingerprint, but we can come pretty close to estimating it with the use of some mathematics…

To start with, we need to work out your Basal Metabolic Rate (or BMR). This is how much energy you would require if you were in a coma.

There are two equations that can be used. Which one to use depends on one thing only; how muscular you are. If you have been going to the gym most of your life and you have above average muscle mass, then use the second equation, called the *Katch McArdle* equation.

If you haven't been hitting the gym, or if you're over 50, then use the first equation. The *Mifflin – St Jeor* equation.

Calculating your BMR using the Mifflin St Jeor Equation:

What you'll need to know:

Body weight (in kg): _____kg

Height (in cm): _____cm

Age (in years): _____years

For males:

BMR = (9.99 x weight) + (6.25 x height) – (4.92 x age) + 5

For females:

BMR = (9.99 x weight) + (6.25 x height) – (4.92 x age) - 161

Just a reminder from school days that the parts in brackets need to be done first.

As an example, let's calculate the BMR for a man who weighs 98kg, is 187cm and 35 year old.

BMR = (9.99 x weight) + (6.25 x height) – (4.92 x age) + 5
BMR = (9.99 x 98kg) + (6.25 x 187cm) – (4.92 x 34yr) + 5
BMR = 979.02 + 1168.75 – 167.28 + 5
BMR = 1,985

Your turn (male):

BMR = (9.99 x weight) + (6.25 x height) – (4.92 x age) + 5
BMR = (9.99 x _____) + (6.25 x _____) – (4.92 x ____) + 5
BMR = (_____) + (_____) – (_____) + 5

My BMR is: _____

(put this in your cheat sheet)

Your turn (female):

BMR = (9.99 x weight) + (6.25 x height) – (4.92 x age) – 161
BMR = (9.99 x _____) + (6.25 x _____) – (4.92 x ____) – 161
BMR = (_____) + (_____) – (_____) – 161

My BMR is: _____

(put this in your cheat sheet)

Calculating your BMR using the Katch McArdle equation:

Remember, only use this equation if you have above average muscle, and you know your body fat percentage. If you'd like to know your body fat percentage, go to the chapter called *How to estimate your body fat percentage*.

What you'll need to know:

Body weight (in kg) _____kg

Body fat percentage: _____%

This calculation has two easy parts. First, you'll need to calculate your lean body mass (LBM). How much you'd weigh without any of your fat on you.

$$LBM = weight - (weight \times bodyfat \div 100)$$

Example, a 64kg person who has 20% body fat:

$LBM = weight - (weight \times bodyfat \div 100)$

$LBM = 64 - (64 \times 20 \div 100)$

$LBM = 64 - 12.8$

$LBM = 51.2 kg$

Your turn:

$LBM = weight - (weight \times bodyfat \div 100)$

LBM = _____ – (_____ x _____ ÷ 100)

LBM = _____ – (_____)

LBM = _____

Now take that answer and plug it into this equation:

$BMR = LBM \times 21.6 + 370$

Using our example before, where we calculated that LBM was 51.2kg:

$BMR = LBM \times 21.6 + 370$

$BMR = 51.2 \times 21.6 + 370$

$BMR = 1,475$

Your turn:

$BMR = LBM \times 21.6 + 370$

BMR = _____ x 21.6 + 370

BMR = _____

MY BMR is _____ calories
(put this on the cheat sheet)

This is how many calories you would use every day if you were in a coma.

How your lifestyle computes

There's way more to your life than being in a coma, right? Well, we can break it down to three things:

- **Exercise Associated Thermogenesis** (EAT). This is the amount of energy burnt during and after exercise. EAT is very often thought to be the biggest factor in fat loss. It's not.

- **Non Exercise Associated Thermogenesis** (NEAT). This is the amount of incidental exercise you do a day, your job, your chores etc. For most people this accounts for far more than EAT, since exercise only lasts about one hour, and you have 24. NEAT accounts for the other 17 waking hours.

- **Thermogenic Effect of Food** (TEF). This is how much energy is required just to digest your food. You want to eat complex foods, like vegetables, because they use up a lot of energy just to be absorbed. Soft drink, on the other hand uses nearly no energy to be absorbed, and has negligible TEF.

We could calculate these individually, but it's much easier and far more practical to just use an estimate. What we call an Activity Factor. Activity factors traditionally combine your lifestyle (NEAT) with your exercise (EAT). But for most adults nowadays, what we do for a job doesn't dictate how active we are outside of work. For this reason, we have split your daily work or career and your exercise.

Circle the number next to your daily non – exercise activity:

	1.0	Desk job/sedentary job
	1.2	Home duties/slightly active (security guard, retail, waitress, chef, personal trainer)
	1.3	Physical job (cleaner, builder, painter)
	1.5	Extremely physical job (bricklayer, landscaper, ski instructor, removalist)

Now circle your level of exercise:

	0	No exercise
	0.1	Light exercise (walking for 30 mins a day)
	0.2	Moderate exercise (30-60 mins intense exercise or sport 3-5 days per week))
	0.4	Lots of exercise (60 mins intense exercise or sport 6-7 days per week)
	0.7	Professional sports person (3-6 hours a day training)

Add the two together to get your activity factor:

_____ + _____ = _____

Lets use an example of a housewife who goes to gym 3 days a week.

$$1.2 + 0.2 = 1.4$$
Activity factor is 1.4

You'll notice that there is a bit of wiggle room between the three bottom rows of exercise. The reason for this is that people's perception of *intense* can be very different to the reality. Intense means that you just could not possibly hold a conversation the entire time. Be honest with yourself here, drop it down a notch if you're not exercising with intensity.

Now, all you have to do to calculate maintenance calories is multiply your activity factor by your BMR which we calculated before. So in the example, the BMR was 1,475 and the activity factor was 1.4.

Maintenance Calories = BMR x Activity Factor
Maintenance Calories = 1475 x 1.4
Maintenance Calories = 2,065

Do yours:

Maintenance Calories = BMR x Activity Factor
Maintenance Calories = _____ x _____

My Maintenance Calories are _____ **Calories**
(put this on the cheat sheet)

You did it, you have calculated how many calories you can eat so that there is no change in your body composition. If you only eat your maintenance calories, you will not gain any more weight. If you eat more than your maintenance calories, you will gain weight. If you eat less than your maintenance calories, you will lose weight!!

It's really that simple.

Note: If you used the first equation, one of the variables is weight, therefore as you lose weight, you should re-evaluate your BMR. You certainly don't need to do it for every kilo lost, but maybe revisit it every time you come down a clothes size.

If you used the second equation, we worked off your LBM, which should not change as you drop fat. You won't need to recalculate your BMR often at all.

Bonus: Breastfeeding

If you're not breastfeeding, skip this chapter.

If you are, then you're giving your baby a lot of energy. Breast milk is very fatty and very sugary. It's true bulking food. Look at how fast a baby develops in the first year. It needs to feed. A newborn needs about 500 calories a day, increasing from there. A 10 month old, weighing around 9kg (20lb) will need around 1,000 calories a day. So if you're a breastfeeding mumma, you need to add in the calories your little food guzzler is using too.

Here's how to calculate how many calories are being lactated…

What you need to know:

How many ml of milk per feed _____
How many feeds per day _____

Once you have written those numbers down, multiply them together, then multiply by 0.7.

For example, a mum knows that she lets down 120ml per feed and she feeds on average 7 feeds in a 24 hour period.

Breastfeeding calories = feed volume x feeds per day x 0.7
Breastfeeding calories = 120 x 7 x 0.7
Breastfeeding calories = 588

Do yours here:

Breastfeeding calories = feed volume x feeds per day x 0.7
Breastfeeding calories = _____ x _____ x 0.7
Breastfeeding calories = _____

Now add that to your maintenance calories that you calculated before. In our example, maintenance calories were 2,065 and breastfeeding calories were 588.

Revised maintenance = maintenance + breastfeeding calories
Revised maintenance = 2,065 + 588
Revised maintenance = 2,653 calories

Do yours:

Revised maintenance = maintenance + breastfeeding Cal
Revised maintenance = _____ + _____
Revised maintenance = _____ calories

My maintenance calories while breastfeeding are _____ calories. *(Put this on the cheat sheet)*

Note: Once you drop a feed, or reduce the volume of milk, you'll need to recalculate this number.

Check it

Now that you've calculated what your maintenance calories should be, we strongly, strongly recommend you check to see if it is accurate. All you have to do is track your calories for 3-7 days to see if it's right. This seems like a tedious task and something you just don't want to do, but it's actually very, very easy.

All you have to do is get an app called *MyFitnessPal* on your phone or computer. Every time you eat something, just put it into the app. If it has a barcode, you just scan the barcode. How easy is that!?! At the end of the day, *MyFitnessPal* will tell you how many calories you ate for the day. At the end of the week, you'll have an enormous insight into your eating habits. Like tracking your spending, it can be one of the most empowering exercises you've ever done.

One thing you need to commit to when using *MyFitnessPal* is to input all food right before you eat it. Not after you ate it, and especially not at the end of the day. Please, please, please input it right before it goes in your mouth. You will be shocked and surprised at what normally goes into your mouth thoughtlessly. If you put the food in later, even with the best intentions, it is nearly impossible to remember everything. Eating for most people is a mindless task, like breathing or going to the toilet.

Can you remember how many breaths you took today, or how many times you went to the toilet, when and where?

How long will it take me?

Here's the fun part. Working out how long it will take you to lose the fat you want to lose. Assuming your maintenance calories are correct, we can calculate how long it will take to get to your goal weight!

Firstly, write down how many kilos you want to lose:

_____kg

Now, write down how long you want to take:

_____weeks

Plug those numbers in here:

    daily deficit = kilos to lose ÷ weeks to take x 1286
    daily deficit = _____ ÷ _____ x 1286
    daily deficit = _____ calories

So lets say our example person wants to lose 5kg in 8 weeks.

> *daily deficit = kilos to lose ÷ weeks to take x 1286*
> *daily deficit = 5 ÷ 8 x 1286*
> *daily deficit = 804 calories*

Once you've calculated your number, just check that it's somewhere below 1000 calories. A deficit of more than 1,000 calories is going to be really hard to maintain. Around 500 calories is really easy to maintain. You barely notice a 500 calorie deficit, but you will notice the weight lost. A 1,000 calorie deficit can feel like a concentration camp. It's up to you though, just work out what you need to do.

Now, to calculate your diet calories, take your calorie deficit number, and subtract it from your maintenance calories.

> *diet calories = maintenance calories – daily deficit*

In our example, we calculated a maintenance of 2,653 calories. We also calculated that to lose 5kg in 8 weeks, she would have to have a deficit of 804 calories. Let's plug all of that into the equation above:

> *diet calories = maintenance calories – daily deficit*
> *diet calories = 2,065 – 804*
> *diet calories = 1,261 calories*

Your turn:

> diet calories = maintenance calories – daily deficit
> diet calories = _____ – _____
> diet calories = _____ calories

Here's another good place to check your numbers. For a female, it's not advisable to go much below 1,200 diet calories, it just becomes more of an exercise in starvation and abstinence than a healthy eating plan. Males, the same goes for you guys below 1,500 calories.

Also, if you are a breastfeeding mother, remember to add in your breastfeeding calories. So in this example, we calculated breastfeeding calories to be 588 calories per day and diet calories to be 1,261 calories per day. The total amount of food that the breastfeeding mum would eat is 1,261 + 588 = 1,849 calories. To maintain the same fat loss after breastfeeding, she'd just revert back to 1,261 calories.

Once you're comfortable with your number above, write it down here:

To lose _____ in _____ weeks, I need to eat _____ calories per day.

Now you have an exact number of calories to eat every single day for however many weeks you wanted, to get to your goal weight! Put the number you calculated into the "diet calories" section of the cheat sheet.

This is the exact calculation the big point-counting companies use. You just got a back door entrance to see the biggest commercial secret in the diet industry. You now have the power to be your own weight loss coach. There are no concepts here, nothing that can be manipulated, just the immutable laws of mathematics. By going through the calculations we just did, you are in the top 1% of people on earth. You know your own numbers.

The freedom you now have, the power…wow!

Your numbers, coupled with entering your food into *MyFitnessPal* means you will never be fooled by your body or by marketing again.

The next part of the book goes into details about what to eat. It is what will allow you to lose fat, without losing muscle, without triggering the starvation response, without dropping your metabolism, and without making you ill or lose energy. In fact the next section is a blueprint for how to gain health and vitality while dieting.

How to estimate your body fat percentage

A lot of what you're about to calculate requires you to know your lean body mass, which is how much you would weigh without any fat on you whatsoever. To do so, we first need to find out what percentage of your body weight is actually fat. There are a few ways to estimate body fat percentage.

The easiest, and least accurate is to hop on a digital body fat scale. If that's all you have, it's accurate enough. It's not the most accurate, but it's certainly accurate enough.

You can go to your doctor and ask for a referral for a DEXA scan. Make sure you tell them you want to calculate your body fat, otherwise they'll calculate your bone density. You could also google DEXA body composition in your area and see what comes up. You'll pay around $80 to get a full, accurate scan.

If you want to do the skin fold tests, then buy a set of skin fold callipers (very cheap) and do a skin fold test. Just follow the instructions that come with the callipers, it's really easy. We use a digital one that cost around $25 on eBay, and it calculates your body fat for you.

The final method is to just eyeball it. We've got a few pictures of body fat percentage for males and females that you can have a look at and compare to on our site here

https://sharnyandjulius.com/how-to-estimate-body-fat/

Whatever method you use, write a number down here:

My Body fat percentage is: _____ %

Another number we're going to need soon is your lean body mass. If you calculated it before, then great, otherwise, here it is:

$$LBM = weight - (weight \times bodyfat \div 100)$$

What you'll need to know:

Bodyweight (in kg) _____ kg

Body fat percentage: _____%

Example, a 64kg person who has 20% body fat:

LBM = weight − (weight x bodyfat ÷ 100)
LBM = 64 − (64 x 20 ÷ 100)
LBM = 64 − 12.8
LBM = 51.2kg

Your turn:

LBM = weight − (weight x bodyfat ÷ 100)
LBM = _____ − (_____ x _____ ÷ 100)
LBM = _____ − (_____)
LBM = _____

My lean Body Mass (LBM) is: _____ kg

Put that number in the front of the book, you'll need it later.

How to prevent muscle loss

Two of the biggest fears people have when dieting are losing muscle, and triggering the starvation response. We'll deal with the starvation response soon, but right now we'll cover how to prevent muscle loss.

Muscle tissue is made up of proteins. Fat and carbohydrates can be stored by the body as body fat and glycogen, but protein cannot be stored. Because muscle is active tissue, it is always breaking down. Generally, people tend to exercise when they diet, so the muscle tissue breaks down even more, since it's being used more. The best way to think of a muscle is to think of a thick rope. The tissue breaking down is like the rope fraying.

To repair the frayed muscle, we need to provide it with enough protein that it can replace the broken down muscle tissue. If we don't eat enough protein, then the muscle just won't get a chance to repair and will deteriorate. It will get weaker and more susceptible to injury. Like the rope, if you fray it too much, some of the bigger fibres could snap or tear. Unlike the rope though, a muscle can repair itself, as long as it has enough amino acids (protein) to do so.

The second reason muscle loss can occur is because during activity, muscles use some amino acids as fuel, specifically and mostly an amino acid called leucine. Because there is no storage for protein, and if there is not enough protein eaten, the muscle will use the leucine that is being used as part of the muscle tissue. Therefore it is important to replace this leucine, and in an ideal situation, eat leucine before exercise so that it is readily available in the blood stream.

Now, here's the important thing though. The loss of muscle described above is not actually visible. Like the frayed rope, it doesn't make the rope look smaller. A muscle is made up of mostly water. 75-79% of a muscle is actually water. So if you think your muscles are shrinking, it's most likely because you are dehydrated, not because your body is eating your muscle like it's a big juicy steak.

Not consuming enough protein over an extended period of time will degrade the muscle to the point that it is noticeable, but it takes a long time. What we're concerned with day to day is keeping the muscles in tip top condition. We want to prevent injury and prevent illness. A steady supply of amino acids (proteins) will do this.

How much is enough?

We've already discovered that proteins can't be stored, so then it would make sense that we eat just enough or just over the protein that is needed. General nutritional guidelines say that you should eat 1g of protein per kilo of lean body weight.

Body composition/ body sculpting / bodybuilding communities tend to agree that 2-3g of protein per kg of lean muscle mass produces the best results for fat loss.

Everybody's needs will be different and you'll be able to tell whether you've got too much. But before we check if you've got too much, let's work out your range.

Take your lean body mass from before (LBM) and write it down here: (it should be on your cheat sheet)

My LBM is _____ kg.

Now just put the number in here:

_____ This is your lower limit of protein intake in grams.

Now, multiply it by 3

_____ x 3 = _____ this is the upper limit of protein intake in grams.

In our example before, the LBM was 51.2kg, so the lower limit of protein intake is 51g, and the upper limit of protein intake is 3 times that. So 51.2 x 3 = 154g (we round the number to make it easier).

The range for protein intake in this example is therefore between 51g and 154g per day. Write your range here:

I should eat somewhere between _____ g and _____ g of protein per day. Don't write this in your cheat sheet, we're going to get an exact figure for you next.

How to tell if you are having too much protein:

We believe that most people eat way too much protein. Both of us have found that 3g per kg of LBM is very high, and we start to show signs of excess.

You will know you've got too much protein in your diet because you will start to stink. Excess protein is broken down with one of the byproducts being ammonia. The stink of someone who is eating too much protein is unbearable. Even sitting in a car with someone can be hard. The cruelest part of this whole dilemma is that the offending person cannot smell themselves.

There is no way to know, other than the honesty of your loving partner, that you smell offensive. And no amount of breath mints or brushing your teeth will fix the burning smell of your breath. If you are dieting and your partner just won't kiss you… drop your protein.

So… avoid the dragon breath and start low. If you don't do much exercise, start at the bottom of your range. If you do a lot of exercise, you'll need to replace more muscle, so start at 2g per kg. In the above example, that would be 51.2 x 2 = 102g per day.

How to tell if you are having too little protein:

You can also tell that you're having too little protein by how sore you are. If you hurt for longer than 3 days after exercise, you may need to increase your protein.

Write down here the number that you feel will be best for you to start with:

_____ g of protein per day. Put this in the cheat sheet at the front of the book.

Now multiply it by 4

_____g of protein x 4 = _____ calories from protein. Put this number in the front of the book as well.

The reason we did the last sum is because each gram of protein accounts for 4 calories of energy. So we can work out how many calories of protein we will eat each day by multiplying our grams of protein by 4.

In our example, the lady is exercising, so we would start at around 2g of protein per kg of LBM. 2g of protein per kg of lean body mass equals 2 x 51.2 = 102g of protein per day. Multiply this by 4 to work out the calories from protein. 102 x 4 = 408 calories from protein.

Remember that her diet calories were 1,849 calories. We can work out what percentage of her diet comes from protein by dividing her diet calories by the calories from protein and multiplying by 100.

percent protein = calories from protein ÷ diet calories x 100
percent protein = 408 ÷ 1,849 x 100
percent protein = 22%

22% of her diet comes from protein

Your turn:

percent protein = calories from protein ÷ diet calories x 100
percent protein = _____ ÷ _____ x 100
percent protein = _____%

Put this number in the front of the book too.

This is another great place to check on your calculations. If your % protein is higher than 50%, you may want to consider dropping your grams of protein per LBM or increasing your diet calories. 50% of your calories from protein is doable, but going over that, in our experience becomes a tough diet health wise. It also becomes a tough diet to stick to. It's totally up to you though, the most important part is that the diet you calculate is sustainable and easy to stick to.

Fats

Fats are important to humans for many reasons. Fats form part of the membrane that surrounds every single cell in the body. Fats also provide the insulating sheath around every single nerve fibre, enabling them to carry messages faster. Vitamins A,D,E and K are fat soluble, not water soluble, so eating fat helps to absorb these important vitamins.

Finally, some of our most important fat loss hormones, such as testosterone, cortisol, oestrogen and progesterone are all made from cholesterol, which is made from fat and protein.

Here's the scoop though – if you need to diet, you already have a lot of fat stored, and ready to be used. You have an abundance of fat. What you don't have is what is called essential fats. Essential fats are fats that the body cannot create from stored fat. You have to get essential fats from the diet.

Based on the above paragraphs, and on the general guidelines that people need to consume around half a gram to 2 gram of fat per kilo of lean muscle mass, we can calculate how much fat you should eat on a daily basis. We want to make sure that hormone production isn't being negatively affected, and we need the essential fats because they play an enormous role in regulating inflammation, cell signaling, reproductive performance and we definitely want to avoid (or reduce) dermatitis (flaky skin).

So, your fat needs are as follows, assuming you have fat to lose:

$$\text{Lower end of fat per day} = LBM \div 2$$
$$\text{Upper end of fat per day} = LBM \times 2$$

In our example, 51.2kg is the LBM, so the fat intake range is:

$$\text{lower end} = 51.2 \div 2 = 26g \text{ of fat}$$
$$\text{upper end} = 51.2 \times 2 = 102g \text{ of fat}$$

26g to 102g of fat, trying to make that up with as much essential fat as possible. Now, as we said before, if you have fat to lose, then you have a good supply on you, so you can afford to eat on the low end of the scale.

Work yours out here:

My LBM is _____ kg

My lower end of fat per day = _____ ÷ 2 = _____ g
My upper end of fat per day = _____ × 2 = _____ g

Right now in the wellness world, there's this huge cry out against a low fat diet, but that is because the low fat diet has been bastardised and commercialized into a high sugar diet. Low fat food tastes plain, and humans are taste driven, not nutrition driven. In order for us to buy low fat food, manufacturers bolstered the flavor by adding sweetness… sugar. Too much sugar, well, too much sugar makes us hungry... or more accurately, gluttonous. This is the only reason low fat has got a bad name.

It makes sense that if you can have a low fat diet, with low sugar, you will get your extra needed fat from your fat stores without becoming gluttonous. The point is not to fall into the conceptual bullshit that a high fat diet is actually good for you. High fat is better than high sugar, just. High fat diets will allow you to lose weight, but the weight will be stored carbohydrates and water. It is true that we don't need nearly as much carbohydrate as the average person eats. This doesn't mean that we have to eat only fat to compensate, though.

While proteins and carbs carry 4 calories per gram, fats carry 9 calories per gram. This means that the more fat you eat, the less carbs and protein you can eat. But it's up to personal preference, as long as you are at the calorie deficit and can sustain it, you will lose fat.

Getting back to the math, we can decide on how much fat we want to consume per day. For us, we like to start at 1g/kg LBM. The reason for this is because it's hard to get the right amount of protein from meat without some fats. We find that limit to be 1g/kg of LBM. Anything below that and a normal, balanced meal becomes all but impossible.

You can go lower in fats, but then you will have to swap meats for protein powders. We find that a bit more fat is actually easier to stick to than a diet that consists of high protein low fat shakes. Just like sugars, they are digested really quickly and don't tend to give you the same feeling of satiety that meat cuts do.

You decide what you want your fat grams to be, remembering to keep it within the range we calculated before. Do it now:

I am going to eat _____ g of fat per day.
(put this on the cheat sheet)

In the example, we would start with 1g/kg of LBM which is smack bang in the middle of the range. Remember that the LBM was 51.2kg. So would look at how 51g of fat would stack up. Just like with protein, we just want to see what percentage of our diet calories will come from fat. Again, anything over 50% is getting too high.

Let's do it for our example first, then you can do yours. Before we do, you need to remember that a gram of fat contains 9 calories, where a gram of protein carries 4 calories. Other than that, the math is essentially the same:

calories from fat = grams of fat x 9
calories from fat = 51 x 9
calories from fat = 459 calories

Your turn:

calories from fat = grams of fat x 9
calories from fat = _____ x 9
calories from fat = _____ calories
(put this on the cheat sheet)

In our example, diet calories was 1,849, so we do the same sum as we did for protein to calculate percent of calories from fat:

percent calories from fat = calories from fat ÷ diet calories x 100
percent calories from fat = 459 ÷ 1,849 x 100
percent calories from fat = 25%

25% of her diet comes from fat

Your turn:

percent fat = calories from fat ÷ diet calories x 100
percent fat = _____ ÷ _____ x 100
percent fat = _____%
(put this on the cheat sheet)

Try to make sure your result is below 50%. If you find that your fat calorie percentage is above 50%, even though you've dropped your fat calories to the lower limit, you may want to go back and increase your diet calories.

Macronutrient balancing

Now that you've worked out your fat and protein, it's a simple calculation to get your carbs. All you have to do, is subtract your fat calories and your protein calories from your diet calories.

Here's the equation we use:

carb calories = diet calories - protein calories - fat calories

In our example, we know that diet calories = 1,849. We also know that protein calories = 408. Finally, we know that fat calories = 459. So let's do the example, then we'll do yours.

carb calories = diet calories - protein calories - fat calories
carb calories = 1849 - 408 - 459
carb calories = 982

Knowing that carbohydrates carry 4 calories per gram, we can just divide by 4 to get the grams of carbs.

grams of carbs = carb calories ÷ 4
grams of carbs = 982 ÷ 4
grams of carbs = 245 grams

Your turn:

> carb calories = diet calories - protein calories - fat calories
> carb calories = _____ - _____ - _____
> carb calories = _____ calories
> (write this in the cheat sheet)

Knowing that carbohydrates carry 4 calories per gram, we can just divide by 4 to get the grams of carbs.

> *grams of carbs = carb calories ÷ 4*
> *grams of carbs = _____ ÷ 4*
> *grams of carbs = _____ g*
> (write this in the cheat sheet)

In our example, diet calories was 1,849, so we do the same sum as we did for protein to calculate percent of calories from carbs:

> *percent carbs = calories from carbs ÷ diet calories x 100*
> *percent carbs = 982 ÷ 1,849 x 100*
> *percent carbs = 53%*

53% of her diet comes from carbs

Your turn:

> *percent carbs = calories from carbs ÷ diet calories x 100*
> *percent carbs = _____ ÷ _____ x 100*

percent carbs = _____%

(put this on the cheat sheet)

If you go back through your working, you can get a ratio of protein, fats and carbs. In this example, we had 22% protein, 25% fat and 53% carbs. You can check that your math is right by adding the percentages, they should add up to 100%. Using this example, 22+25+53=100.

Write your ratios here:

Protein _____%
Fats   _____%
Carbs _____%

Add them together: _____ + _____ + _____ = _____

If your percentages add up to 100, you've done your math right! If they are close, as in 99% or 101%, that's fine too - it's a rounding thing and not important. Just add or subtract a percentage point off the carbs.

Now that you've gotten to this step, you should have almost all of your cheat sheet filled in. On the following page is what the cheat sheet would look like for our example.

Cheat Sheet

Weight loss goal __**5**__ kg

Weeks to lose weight __**8**__ weeks

Maintenance calories __**2,653***__ calories

Lean Body Mass (LBM) __**51.2**__ kg

Diet calories __**1,849***__ calories

Protein __**102**__ grams __**408**__ calories __**22**__ %

Fats __**51**__ grams __**459**__ calories __**25**__ %

Carbs __**245**__ grams __**982**__ calories __**53**__ %

Carb refeed _____ grams _____ calories

*includes breastfeeding calories

How to eat whatever you want

Now that you have your framework, you can eat anything you want at all, as long as if fits within your calories and macros. To check this, just input your diet calories and macros into the goals section of *MyFitnessPal*.

You may have to round the percentages to the nearest 5. To do so, you'll need to take from one macro and give to another. As a general rule, we would take from carbs to give to the other 2 macros. So using our example, we have

Protein	22%
Fat	25%
Carbs	53%

As you can see, fats are already rounded to the nearest 5, but protein and carbs aren't. So we'd round protein up to 25%, and carbs down to 50%. You can check that you've rounded correctly by adding your new numbers together. As long as they add up to 100%, you're on track.

The numbers we'd put into the goals section of *MyFitnessPal* would therefore be:

Calories: 1,849
Protein: 25%
Fat: 25%
Carbs: 50%

You may have to input your macros and calories to the goals section manually, so bypassing the automatic calculation by *MyFitnessPal*. You definitely want to do this.

Once you've added your goals, simply log everything you eat, and make sure that it fits within your macros and calorie goals. *MyFitnessPal* will tell you if you've gone over by turning the result at the bottom of the table into red text.

This is essentially the basis of flexible dieting, or "if it fits your macros" (IIFYM). Many fitness models subscribe to this theory, and as far as body composition goes, they are great testament to the fact that it doesn't matter what you eat, as long as it fits your macros.

The classic example is a McChicken Burger, which has exactly the same macros as brown rice and tuna. 25g protein, 33g carbs and 15g fat.

How exciting is that!

You could literally put the book down right now and be better off than 99.9% of the population. You should give yourself a pat on the back, because you've worked through some serious math to find out exactly what your own numbers are. You've saved yourself a ton of money by avoiding the commercial diets and a ton of stress by avoiding conceptual diets.

There is a bit more to cover, and we promise that it will be illuminating. So stick with us, we guarantee you'll be pumped, especially when we get to the refeed section!

Prioritise health

While you could live off McDonalds and icecream and still get your body composition goals, there is so much more to food than calories and macros. One thing we can take from conceptual diets is that we need to prioritise health.

We know that body composition is not the only marker of health. It is a broad one, but certainly not all encompassing. If you're obese, then there is a very high chance you are also unhealthy, but if you're ripped with a 6 pack, it doesn't mean you are healthy. In fact, the 6 pack guy is far more susceptible to shock death, because his physique lures him into a false sense of health. Thinking you can eat whatever you want because you look healthy is very dangerous.

Speed addicts are a great example of this. They may look lean and ripped and healthy to the naked eye, but we all know that they are in fact dying inside, slowly destroying their organs and their nervous system.

We have always maintained that if you are not proactive about your health, you will succumb to the environment that you live in. Unfortunately for almost all of us, that environment is geared toward convenience and consumption. Convenience comes at a cost of quality.

Compare yourself to a car. For a car to be repaired, the mechanic removes the old part, and bolts on a brand new one, made from good quality materials at a factory with good quality control measures. The part comes from outside of the car.

For a human to repair itself, we get spare parts from one place only, and that is our food. If you feed yourself junk, you'll be made up of junk. If you feed yourself good quality, nutrient dense food, you'll be made up of good quality nutrient dense cells.

This is what we mean, when we say prioritise health. By all means, eat some entertainment food once in a while, make sure it fits your macros, but don't be fooled into believing that you can survive off it forever.

Along with the calories, comes nutrition. Over processed food contains barely any nutrition. In fact, the nutrition has often been stripped out and replaced with poisons, such as preservatives, additives and colours.

This is where your conceptual diet plays a big part. At the beginning of the book, we said to keep your conceptual diet in your back pocket.

Now's the time to bring it out. Conceptual diets prioritise health, so plug your concept into your framework and you've got a diet that will actually make you healthier while predictably and consistently facilitating fat loss.

How to lose the first few kilos really fast

Many diets promise fast results. "We guarantee that you will lose 5kg in the first week or your money back." Who doesn't want to lose 5kg in the first week? What a guarantee, I've basically got no risk - where do I sign up?

You and I both know that those first 5 kilos are definitely not all fat. This is what we hate about our industry and why we have written this book. The diet industry is plagued by cowboys and profiteers who prey on your desperation for fast results. The greasy prick who stands in front of you telling you that you can lose 5 kilos in the first week is not lying, but he's certainly not being honest either. That slimy salesman is not interested in helping you, he's interesting in his own wallet.

Here's the truth. In the first week of any diet, you will very likely lose a lot more weight than you expected. Especially if you are man. Unfortunately for women, there is a chance that you can actually gain weight. It all depends on your water retention.

Carbohydrates, especially fruits and vegetables contain a lot of water and a lot of fibre. The fibre sits in your digestive tract and weighs around 2 kilos at any one time. Your body is made up of mostly water, which can fluctuate by 5 kilos at any one time.

One of the fastest ways to drop weight (not necessary fat) is to reduce your carbohydrates to near zero. After a few days you'll have crapped out all the fibre, and by eating mostly protein, you would have been eating a diuretic. A diuretic forces your body to flush out a lot of water, essentially dehydrating you. It is quite common to lose 5-8kg of fluid in the first week.

You feel like you're losing weight, which is the only good thing, but a double edged sword. If you lose weight that fast, why not wait another week, enjoy the junk food for a bit, it will only take a week to lose 5 kilos after all, right?

Fat is stored in the body anhydrously (without water). Carbs are stored in the body with water. So for every gram of carbohydrate, there are an additional 2g of water. If you use up say, 1kg of carbs in a week, you will lose that 1kg of carbs and 2kg of water (3kg of weight, none of which is fat). You may be lighter, but you'll still be fat.

One thing you can expect is that for most people quitting junk food, there is a relatively large flushing of inflammation. Think about the last time you saw a rolled ankle. It was swollen. It wasn't fat, even though it looked fat, it was just inflamed. Inflammation is mostly water. The water is packed in tight to protect the damaged joint.

If you've been eating junk, there is a good chance that you have inflammation throughout your body. It's like a small allergic reaction every time you eat. A few days after eating the last piece of offending food, your body flushes out the inflammation, assuming that the threat is gone. This is not fat loss, it is a reduction in inflammation. But unlike the high protein diet, it is loss of unnecessary water. The water and carbs you lose in the high protein, low carb diet need to come back. The inflammation reduction is permanent.

For many people the inflammation is actually in the skin, making a person look fat. To lose the inflammation is more remarkable, and better for you than losing the fat. Simply eating for *health* will do this. Don't fall trap to the greasy salesmen who tell you that high protein, low carbs will make you lose fat. It's like not paying your bills so that you look like you have lots of money.

How to never be hungry

Forget about what macronutrient gives you the best feeling of satiety, nothing can curb hunger better than a stomach filled with food.

Too often, dieters find themselves constantly hungry. While hunger can be a good sign that your body is tapping into fat stores, and can be worn as a badge of honour, we believe it to be unnecessary.

When we create a food plan for someone, the first priority after balancing calories and macros, is to ensure that the volume of food is so high that the person struggles to finish each meal.

There are a few tricks that we use to achieve this, but before we get into those, think about the diets you've been on where food was basically reduced to small portions, and you always had this feeling that you were being deprived.

We're willing to bet that that feeling alone accounts for most people quitting on a diet. Followed immediately by a binge of epic proportions and the inescapable feeling of failure. Don't worry, we've all been there. The good news is you don't have to ever again. With the following tricks, you'll never starve yourself again.

Eat food that is harder to digest.

Part of the reason people gain body fat is that the calories consumed are just so easily obtained from the food. Satiety, the feeling of content, "I'm not hungry anymore" is primarily dictated by fullness of the belly. Drinking soft drink, laden with calories, seems to the body to be just like water, and unrecognizable as a food source. Drinking 600ml of coke gives 258 calories, but no feeling of being full. To get the same amount of energy from a garden salad would require 1.5kg of salad.

Do you think you could even eat 1.5kg of salad in one sitting? 1.5kg of salad contains so much more than just calories and carbs. The micronutrients in that would make your body sing to you!!

Many people who eat what we recommend report that they just can't eat that much food. See, before they were eating less volume but more calories. Now, they're eating more volume, but less calories. The remaining volume is where all the good stuff is stored!

Vegetables are phenomenal for this. Most people are used to eating rice or pasta to *fatten out* their meals. We grate or blend cauliflower to replace rice and we spiral zucchini to replace spaghetti. You cannot tell the difference, even though cauliflower has 1/5th of the calories that rice has, and zucchini has 1/10th of the calories that spaghetti has. How cool is that!!

The same goes for protein sources. We prefer that you get your daily protein requirements from solid food than from liquid. Protein shakes do not make you feel full the way chicken breast does.

Avoid lunches with friends.

At around mid morning, people tend to be really, really hungry (for good reason). But we put off eating with a coffee and a snack, then have a huge lunch.

We recommend that you eat a proper meal when you're hungry (mid morning) and use the lunch break (if you get one) to go for a walk. You'll notice that you will skip the mid afternoon slump, and you'll avoid the lunch rush, as well as the smell of everyone else's fatty, greasy, fast food lunches.

Early afternoon, when everyone else is starting to crash, you'll have another proper meal. Still light in comparison to theirs, but you'll be able to power through the rest of your day until your early dinner. Productivity will be up, and you'll be better equipped to do something at night other than lying on the couch!

Reduce the glycemic load

Most people believe that carbs are just sugars, breads, pastas and rices. But what most people don't know is that fruits and vegetables are carbohydrates too. In fact, technically, fibre is a carbohydrate. It may be undigested in the small intestine, but the bacteria in the large intestine digest it, and for want of a better explanation, poo it out in a form that our body can use as fuel. So even fibre carries with it a carbohydrate load.

Which brings about an interesting point. We can only use a certain amount of carbohydrate at a time. If we overload the system by eating too many carbohydrate calories at once, our body responds by storing it as fat. Fructose, the carbohydrate found in fruit as well as most processed foods, is stored very easily, as it is processed by the liver and turned into fat. This is important to know. Fructose (a type of sugar) is easily turned into fat.

We don't include fruits in our meal plans at all. Fruits have become a little bit too much like a fructose bomb. Through the miracles of modern science and food technology, we've got super-sweet fruit that is 10 to 100 times sweeter than the original fruit it once was.

There are exceptions, however. Bananas are a magical fruit that are more of a resistant starch than a carbohydrate – as part of a balanced diet, we like to include a resistant starch. Bananas are cheap, easy and tasty.

Granny Smith apples are high in pectin, which helps to slow the release of insulin – apples are a great low GI snack that you can carry with you anywhere. Carry apples, not grapes. Grapes are little sugar bombs. Try it for yourself some time. Try to stop at about 10 grapes… go on… do it!!

In this diet, we recommend that you account for your carb intake by using vegetables. Vegetables don't spike your blood sugar and therefore won't cause insulin spikes. Insulin is an essential hormone, but very dangerous in high concentration. Many modern diseases can be attributed to elevated levels of insulin. The fastest way to increase insulin is to consume high GI (sweet) foods. So we reduce the insulin impact by eating low GI foods (vegetables). After a little while you will get used to it, and you won't be on the blood sugar roller coaster any more. The tired/wired/tired/wired feeling will just flatten out.

Reduce the booze

Under normal conditions, your body gets its energy from the calories in carbohydrates, fats and proteins. To release these calories, the food needs to be digested, which uses energy. Even dextrose, the simplest digestible carbohydrate, needs some digestion.

Alcohol, on the other hand requires no digestion. It simply slips straight through the stomach to the small intestine, where it jumps the queue ahead of your normal food, straight to the blood stream. Once in the blood stream, your liver works very hard to rid your system of this poison, which means that there is no attention paid to the other foods in the blood. These carbohydrates and fats are therefore stored for later – as body fat.

Because there is no food in the body, you feel really hungry as soon as you stop drinking. For some of us, we feel hungry even while we're drinking, and we're never hungry for a salad. It's always the greasy, fatty crap late night food merchants sell.

While this is going on, the function of your kidneys has been distracted. Your kidneys are a blood filter – they catch all the nasty stuff in your blood (which is suspended in water). All the nasties are passed out as urine, and the water is put back into the blood stream on the other side. When alcohol is in the blood, your kidneys just pass everything out as urine – nasties, alcohol and water. This is why a hangover feels like dehydration – it is dehydration.

All of this work affects the liver in some horrible ways. Being the biggest internal organ, it plays a key role in the major functions of the human body. Cirrhosis of the liver occurs when good, healthy organ tissue is replaced with bad scar tissue, due to constant overexposure to alcohol. This bad tissue then keeps the liver from having blood flow through, which in turn stops it from working properly.

If that's not bad enough, alcohol consumption prior to sleep reduces the quality of your sleep. Not only do you have to get up to urinate, but your body will only allow you deep, reparative sleep once the alcohol has been fully metabolised – one hour per standard drink. This means that if you were to have 6 beers before bed, you would not begin your deep sleep for 6 hours, which means in the morning, you feel as though you have only had 2 hours of sleep.

Interesting fact: the calories contained in one can of beer will take 42 minutes to walk off. That means to burn off a 6 pack of beer would take 4 hours and 15 minutes of walking – if that's all you had. Or, you could just run a half marathon.

Avoid starvation mode

Because you are reducing your calories below maintenance, your body will respond by downregulating non-essential processes. Things such as hair growth, reproduction, general energy etc. What this does is make your calorie needs actually drop.

To combat this, we need to incorporate a refeed meal once or twice a week. Basically a refeed meal is a way to trick your body into believing that it is getting a surplus of calories. What happens is that it then doesn't downregulate your metabolism, instead increasing it so that over the next few days, you lose even more fat. Right before the body starts to slow things down again, we do another refeed.

Now a refeed is NOT a free for all binge. You can (and should) eat up to your calculated maintenance on the day of your refeed, but anything above that will be stored, so be warned – the purpose of the refeed is to stoke the fire, not have a full on food orgy.

We also warn that a refeed should contain only carbs and protein, not fat. Having carbs and fats in surplus is a sure fire way to ensure that the fat eaten is stored.

How much to eat on a refeed:

This will be your final calculation in the Math diet. All you have to do is to ensure that you eat up to your maintenance calories on your refeed day. If you regularly eat 4 meals a day, on your refeed day, eat a fifth meal, comprised mostly of carbohydrates.

To calculate how much, simply subtract your diet calories from your maintenance calories.

refeed calories = maintenance calories – diet calories

In our example, the maintenance was 2,653 calories and the diet calories were 1,849.

refeed calories = maintenance calories – diet calories
refeed calories = 2,653 – 1,849
refeed calories = 804

You'll notice that the refeed works out to be exactly the same as the deficit we calculated.

Your turn:

>refeed calories = maintenance calories − diet calories
>refeed calories = _____ − _____
>refeed calories = _____
>
>*(put this in your cheat sheet)*

Now, simply divide by 4 to see how many grams of carbs you can add to your refeed day.

>*grams of carbs = refeed calories ÷ 4*

In our example,

>*Refeed carbs = refeed calories ÷ 4*
>*Refeed carbs = 804 ÷ 4*
>*Refeed carbs = 201g of carbs.*

We originally calculated that the allowable carbs were 245g, so on a carb refeed day, we're nearly doubling the carb intake. When we design custom food plans for people, we ensure that you struggle to eat all the food on a diet day, so on a refeed day, you'll need to eat higher GI carbs just so that you can actually fit them all in.

Great carb sources are brown rice, rolled oats, bananas, sweet potatoes, quinoa and potatoes. If you're not averse to wheat, you can add in breads or pastas.

Your turn:

    Refeed carbs = refeed calories ÷ 4
    Refeed carbs = _____ ÷ 4
    Refeed carbs = _____ g of carbs.
    (put this in your cheat sheet)

When to refeed:

Step 1: Buy ketostix from the chemist

Step 2: Pass a stick through your urine after every meal. Don't worry, they're actually really cheap.

Step 3: When you see any sign of colour change on the ketone scale for 2 meals in a day, add a refeed meal to the very next day.

Step 4: Repeat steps 2 and 3!

Obviously we all diet because we are carrying too much fat, which is felt as excess weight. There is only really one way to lose body fat and that is to reduce calorie intake. But, as we said before, that comes with a cost – a delayed onset of metabolic downregulation. This is why you MUST do the refeed days and do them properly. Be patient, you will gain weight on your refeed day, but that is because the muscles and liver are restocking glycogen, not because of storing fat. The process kind of looks like this:

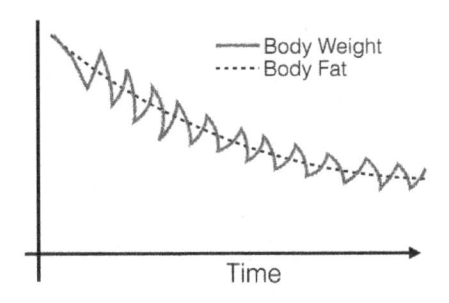

So your weight will go up and down like a yo-yo, but the overall body fat will reduce gradually, because your weekly calories are below maintenance.

Increase your metabolism

The holy grail of body composition. Eating more than you did when you were fat, but maintaining a lean and toned physique.

Unfortunately there is no food you can eat that will speed up your metabolism significantly. Some foods may cause you to burn slightly more energy, but the increase is very, very slight. Caffeine on the other hand is a central nervous system (CNS) stimulant that studies have shown to increase BMR by 3% - 11%. This is not a bad result. Using an example BMR of 1500 calories, that means caffeine can increase BMR by 45 to 165 calories. At 45 calories, you would lose a kilo of fat in 7 months. If you're on the higher end, that would be a kilo on under 8 weeks. Not too shabby for a cuppa.

Caffeine also blunts your appetite, as well as a host of other fat loss benefits, and is why almost every fat loss supplement or pre workout drink contains caffeine. Just be careful of having too much caffeine - read the label and compare to your current tolerance. Instant coffee has 31mg of caffeine per teaspoon. No Doz tablets contain 100mg. Some pre workouts contain 200-300mg. 300mg is nearly 10 cups of coffee. That's a lot of caffeine!

The problem with taking such high doses is that your body very quickly adapts to the stimulant effects. If you take a pre workout of 300mg, then the next day, your regular coffee is just not going to cut it anymore. After a week or so, the 300mg is not going to give you the same effect, which is when most people double the dose!

The smartest way to caffeinate yourself is to cycle it. 2 weeks on, one week off. That way you can keep your doses at safe levels, and still enjoy the fat burning benefits.

Some people will tell you that gaining muscle will increase metabolism. Studies have shown that an increase of every 1kg of muscle translates to about 12 calories per day increase in metabolism, which is negligible.

What does drive the metabolism through the roof is *rebuilding* damaged muscle. Weight training breaks down muscle tissue which requires huge amounts of energy and amino acids to repair. If the weight is heavy enough, the CNS will stimulated as well, giving a short term (8hr - 48hr) increase in BMR.

Talking about CNS stimulation, lower intensity cardio has shown to have a negligible effect on fat loss. The reason being that the body adapts to, and becomes very efficient at low intensity cardio. High intensity cardio performed to exhaustion has a much better effect on your CNS and therefore your maintenance calories over the next day or two. It also takes less time than steady state cardio.

But here's the thing about exercise, you've got to stimulate the CNS to get the increase in metabolism after the exercise is complete. If you finish your workout feeling fresh, then your metabolism will return to normal within an hour. If you are laying on the ground, struggling to even breathe after a workout, or if you feel like you just want to go to sleep right where you finished your workout, then the metabolism will be ramped up for 24 to 48 hours.

So, there is no permanent way to increase your metabolism, or your maintenance calories other than getting a more physical job. If you're a stay at home mum or dad, why not become more active by playing with your kids, or taking them for walks.

To give you an example of the benefits of this, have a look at our online programs for mums and dads. Participants have increased their metabolisms so much, just by playing with their kids that they have lost upwards of 10 kilos of fat in only an 8 week period. Exercise doesn't have to be restricted to the gym - it can be done with your family. To you it's exercise, to them it's play. Play that they will remember for their entire lives.

Sport is another great example of exercise that is fun. If you have the time, join a social sports team. The camaraderie and the competitiveness will have you doing high intensity interval training without you even realising it.

Putting it all together

While it's fun to just eat whatever you want as long as it fits within your macros, we all could do with a bit more structure in our lives. Eating whatever, whenever is part of the reason most of us became fat in the first place.

To save time, and to give yourself even more chance at success, we recommend you create a meal plan for yourself. Be proactive with *MyFitnessPal* rather than reactive. Put your meals in *before* you eat them, rather than after.

To give you even more chance of success, we recommend you create a meal plan that fits your macros and calories for only one day. Simple is better than complicated. When we heard that The Rock ate the same meals every single day for 6 months, we thought "what a ridiculously clever idea!"

You see, habits are built through repetition. If you eat the same meals every day, healthy eating will become a habit. When you break that habit by eating something out of the ordinary, you will notice it. It won't be mindless and it won't go unnoticed.

Secondly, when most people fall off the bandwagon, they wait until Monday to start the diet again. If you eat the same food every day, that means you can get back on the bandwagon the very next day, limiting the damage and laying down repetition and habits that will have you looking lean and toned before you know it.

Remember that losing fat takes time, and because of the Math Diet, you've even worked out how much time. Consistency and patience are very, very important to you achieving your dream body. Eating the same meals every day will go a long way to creating consistency... then all you need to work on is your patience.

Just remember that if you start today, you'll get there a day sooner than if you start tomorrow.

We know that creating the eating plan that fits your macros and calories, while prioritising health and keeping you from hunger is time consuming work. It's rewarding, but it does take time, so if you want us to do the work for you, head here:

https://sharnyandjulius.com/personalised-meal-plan/

We will calculate your calorie and macro needs, then create a customised food plan based on your food likes and dislikes, as well as make the meals delicious, easy to cook and healthy.

We'll even include some delicious, filling carb refeed options, so you can get to your dream body with ease. Before you know it, you'll be there!

Talk to us!

We'd love to hear from you, please let us know if and how this book has helped you. Just shoot us a quick email at

sharnyandjulius@sharnyandjulius.com

Thankyou for taking the time to read our book!

Sharny and Julius Kieser

You can also follow us on social media by searching:

sharnyandjulius

The Kiesers

527 kids
1 Parent = 12 kids

527 ÷ 12 = 12
          6 2

```
    0 8 4 r2
6 ) 5̶5̶ 2̶ 47
```